A Doctor in your Suitcase

*Natural medicine for self-care
when you are away from home.*

By
Dr. Michael Gazsi
Naturopathic Physician
and
Nina Anderson, S.P.N.

A Doctor in your Suitcase
by Dr. Michael Gazsi & Nina Anderson

ISBN 0-9701110-2-9
Library of Congress Catalog Card Number 00-133651
Categories: 1.Health   2. First Aid   3. Medicine
4.Travel 5. Homeopathy 6. Herbal

Printed in North America

Edited by Cherie Tripp

A Doctor In Your Suitcase is not intended as medical advice. It is written solely for informational and educational purposes. Please consult a health professional should the need for one be indicated. Because there is always some risk involved, the authors and publisher are not responsible for any adverse effects or consequences resulting from the use of any of the suggestions, preparations or methods described in this book. The publisher does not advocate the use of any particular diet or health program, but believes that the information presented in this book should be available to the public.

Published by New Century Publishers 2000

Canadian office:	US office:
60 Bullock Dr. Unit 7	283 East Canaan Rd.
Markham ON LP3 3P2	East Canaan, CT 06024
(905) 471-7885	(860) 824-5301

Introduction

You will find this book a welcome addition to your travel needs, particularly if you are trying to avoid chemical or pharmaceutical first aid treatments. This text will help you find useful and concise information with ease, when it is needed. *A Doctor in your Suitcase* will help the reader know what remedies should be on hand, while traveling.

Illness often occurs when you are away from home. The motto "be prepared" advises us to have the basic natural products available for the proper treatment of acute conditions. When a patient calls or pages a health care practitioner, those who have the needed products at home will most likely, find the fastest relief.

Using This Book

Each ailment has several types of treatment options represented. These are categorized as nutrition, herbal medicine, homeopathic medicine, and home remedies. You will find many remedies offered which are safer, less invasive, non-intrusive and non-toxic. Many can be tried first, before resorting to prescription medication. Information in this book enables you to handle minor ailments or injuries yourself, but it is not intended to replace your physician. This book can help you become knowledgeable about all treatment options if medical intervention is indicated, so that you and your physician can work as a team. All dosages recommended are for adults, unless indicated.

A few words of caution: if you are currently being treated for a specific condition, consult your health-care practitioner before trying any of the recommended remedies in this book. Do not discontinue current prescription medications without consulting your physician.

The remedies in this book have an established history of safe use. However, even natural remedies may cause reactions, especially in very sensitive or ill individuals, or when not used properly.

Maintaining a natural first-aid kit while traveling will pay off as health emergencies arise. You can assemble kit components yourself, or purchase ready-made kits that are becoming more readily available *(see product manufacturers in Appendix)*.

Dosage amounts recommended in the book are intended for adults, unless indicated otherwise. Multiple remedies may be recommended. To our knowledge, there have been no complications nor side-effects when taking any remedy in combination with another listed remedy. Homeopathic remedies may be negated by strong stimulants such as black tea, excessive amounts of chocolate, camphor, coffee, mint and strong odors such as garlic. If you find an interaction occurring when taking multiple remedies simultaneously, seek advice from a licensed health-practitioner.

Women who are pregnant or nursing should never begin any self-care remedies without working closely with their health care professional. Before you begin using natural remedies, always discuss your intended use with your health care provider. If an acute illness becomes prolonged, always seek the guidance of a professional.

+For standard emergency action principles, such as techniques for choking, rescue breathing, treating wounds, bites, sprains and CPR, please refer to handbooks and courses offered by the American Red Cross. They also supply information about preparing your accessories such as bandages, gauze, butterfly closures, etc.

The "away-from-home"
Basic Natural-Medicine Kit

Components:

Herbal:

Aloe gel
(topical anti-infective)   (pg. 11)

Echinacea, goldenseal
(internal herbal antibiotic)   (pg. 20, 21, 72)

Ginger
(Motion sickness, diarrhea)   (pg. 36, 66)

Aged Garlic extract
(topical herbal antiseptic)   (pg. 27)

White willow
(Natural aspirin)   (pg. 45)

Homeopathic:

Arnica
(Pain relief)   (pg. 25, 44, 82)
Natrum. Mur   (pg. 14, 23, 47, 55)
(insect bites, colds, headache, indigestion)

Flower remedy:

First-aid remedy (also known as rescue remedy or five-flower remedy)
(emotional trauma, shock, terror)   (pg. 16. 31. 84)

In addition, we recommend adding gauze, cotton balls, and bandages to your kit.

Table of Contents

BITES/STINGS

Quick Reference:

Nutritional Care:
Vitamin C

Herbal:
Aloe vera
Black Salve
Calendula
Echinacea
Plantain

Homeopathic:
Apis 12C or 30C
Lachesis 6C
Ledum 3OC
Natrum Mur, 6X
Stapysagria 12C

Home Remedies:
Baking soda
First Aid Flower remedy
Soap

Treatment Details:

Warning: *These remedies cannot exempt one from allergic reactions to bee stings, which can include fainting and difficulty breathing. Seek help from a medical professional without delay, if you experience these symptoms.*

Nutritional Care	*Bites & Stings*

+Vitamin C
Properties: Vitamin C can decrease reactivity to stings, as well as reduce swelling and pain.
Dosage: 1000 mg 3-4 times per day with meals.

+ **Aloe vera gel**

Properties: This gel works to draw the stinger out. Aloe promotes tissue healing and prevents infections. It may create a burning sensation in the affected area. This means it is working.

External application: Extracted from the aloe plant, aloe gel can be applied 4-6 times daily. You can also break off a piece of an aloe plant and rub the sticky plant gel on your wound.

+ **Black Salve or ointment**

Herbal preparation of bloodroot, galangal, red clover, and sheep sorrell. Can be purchased already formulated.

Properties: This salve works to draw the stinger out. It may create a burning sensation in the affected area. This means it is working.

External application: Smear enough salve to cover area of sting.

+ **Calendula**

Properties: Speeds healing and reduces infection.

External application: Apply 4-6 times daily.

Available in an oil or cream, calendula should be applied externally after a wound has closed and risk for infection is past.

+ **Echinacea root**

Properties: Traditionally used for the treatment of animal bites, including snake bites.

Dosage: 50 drops of liquid extract in 4 oz. warm water, as required.

External application: A poultice of dry or fresh root may be applied externally as well.

+ **Plantain poultice**.

Properties: Found commonly in and around our yards, plantain is used to treat insect bites and stings.

External application: Prepare as follows: Chop fresh herb and place in blender with a little water. Puree to make a thick paste. Spread on gauze and apply to bite or sting. Keep moist. Repeat as required. When hiking or camping and blender is not available, chew fresh plantain and apply mash to affected area.

Homeopathic remedies may be negated by strong stimulants such as black tea, excessive amounts of chocolate, camphor, coffee, mint and strong odors such as garlic.

Choose from the following remedies, depending on the type of bite you are suffering from. Strength of remedy (12C, 6X) will be indicated on supplement.

+ Apis 12C or 30C
Properties: Red, inflamed insect bites or stings that cause burning sensation and pain.
Dosage: 5 pellets dissolved under the tongue every 15 to 60 minutes, until symptoms stop increasing, then 5 pellets 2 to 4 times daily until the symptoms subside.

+ Lachesis 6C
Properties: Bites from a dog, tarantula, or leeches.
Dosage: 5 pellets dissolved under the tongue every 15-60 minutes until symptoms stop increasing, then 5 pellets 2-4 times per day until the symptoms subside.

+ Ledum 3OC

Properties: Relieves symptoms resulting from the bites or stings of mosquitoes, bees, wasps, scorpions, spiders, rats and angry animals.

Dosage: 5 pellets dissolved under the tongue every 15-60 minutes until symptoms stop increasing, then 5 pellets 2-4 times per day until the symptoms subside.

External application: Moisten skin, dissolve pellets in water and apply directly to wound.

+ Natrum Mur 6X

Properties: <u>The primary cell salt remedy for insect bites.</u>

Dosage: 5 pellets dissolved under the tongue every 15 to 60 minutes until symptoms stop increasing, then 5 pellets 2 to 4 times daily until the symptoms subside.

External application: Moisten skin, dissolve pellets in water and apply directly to wound.

+ Stapysagria 12C

Properties: Effective against mosquito or other insect bites that are extremely itchy and raise large welts.

Dosage: 5 pellets dissolved under the tongue every 15-60 minutes until symptom stops increasing, then 5 pellets 2-4 times per day until the symptoms subside.

+ Baking soda
Properties: Draws out the stinger and neutralizes the acidic bee venom.
External application: Mix with a little water to make a paste, and apply directly to the sting.

+ First Aid Flower Remedy (cherry plum, clematis, impatiens, rock rose, and Star of Bethlehem)
Properties: Gives relief and healing during and following emergencies, accidents, shock, injury, insect and animal bites or any trauma or terror.
Dosage: 3 drops orally under the tongue in 5-10 minute intervals as needed.

+ Soap
External application: Immediately after an insect sting, grab a bar of soap and run it over the sting area. Soap seems to have an affinity for stingers and will draw them out, preventing further infection from the venom.

Quick Reference:

Nutritional Care:
Vitamin C
Ionized silver
Trace minerals
Velvet antler
Zinc

Herbal:
Aged Garlic Extract
Cold care tea
Echinacea
Goldenseal
Rhododendron caucasicum

Homeopathic:
Aconitum 6C
Arsenicum 6C
Bryonia 6C
Ferrum phos. 6X
Natrum mur. 6X
Pulsatilla 6C
Rus tox 6C

Home Remedies:
Diet
Green tea

Treatment Details:

Nutritional Care	*Colds/flu*

+ **Vitamin C**
Properties: Antiviral and antibacterial. Strengthens host resistance.
Dosage: 1,000 to 3000 mg every day. Slowly cut back to normal levels after cold or acute disorder has subsided.

+ **Ionized silver**
Properties: An effective non-toxic bacteria-killing substance. Ionization reduces silver to its smallest particle (homeopathic preparation) for increased absorption, with reduced side-effects.
Dosage: 1 tablespoon (from solution of 10 ppm diluted in 16 oz. water) in 8 oz. water daily. Take for 10 days maximum (similar to an antibiotic).

+ **Trace Minerals**
Properties: "Jump starts" the immune system to fight cold virus.
Dosage: (Liquid electrolyte solutions) Take 1 tsp. in 8 oz. of water every 15 minutes for 4 hours, then 3 times per day thereafter. (Capsules) Take as recommended on specific bottle.

+ Velvet Antler
Properties: From antlers harvested humanely from elk. Use for recovery from respiratory infections.
Dosage: As per instructions on the supplement bottle. Normal dosage is 1-3 capsules per day.

+ Zinc (if over 14 years of age)
Properties: Good for sore throat.
Dosage: 50 mg of elemental zinc from amino acid chelate taken with meals, or suck on zinc lozenges containing 23 mg of elemental zinc every two hours while awake. Do not use lozenges this frequently for more than one week.

+ Aged Garlic extract
Properties: Powerful antibiotic and antiviral.
Dosage: 1 to 2 capsules every two hours of standardized aged garlic extract, until cold dissipates. Fresh, raw garlic, a whole, living food, is acceptable. Eat two chopped cloves of garlic at first sign of cold.
Note: Raw parsley taken with raw garlic will help prevent "garlic breath" and enhance garlic's blood cleansing effects.

+ Cold care tea (elder-flowers, peppermint, yarrow, cat's claw)
Properties: Traditional formula for resolving colds and flu. (promotes perspiration)
Preparation: Use a heaping teaspoonful of the herbal combination per 8-oz. pure water. Steep for 30 minutes and strain. Drink freely throughout the day.

+ Echinacea
Properties: Antiviral and an immune stimulant.
Dosage: 2 to 4 capsules, or 50 drops of liquid extract 3 to 4 times daily for two weeks.
Note: It is important to begin at first sign of cold.

+ Goldenseal

Properties: Antiviral and an immune stimulant.

Dosage: 2 to 4 capsules or 40 to 50 drops of liquid extract three times daily for up to 14 days. Take in combination with echinacea.

Note: Decrease dosage if nauseated.

+ Rhododendron caucasicum

Properties: One of the most powerful antioxidants in the world. Helps to prevent spread of infection.

Dosage: 3 capsules per day.

Homeopathic remedies may be negated by strong stimulants such as black tea, excessive amounts of chocolate, camphor, coffee, mint, and strong odors such as garlic.

Choose from the following remedies, depending on the type of cold symptom you are suffering from. Strength of remedy (12C, 6X) will be indicated on supplement.

+ **Aconitum 6C**
Properties: Used primarily during the first 24-hour onset period of a cold or flu. Sudden onset of fever with chills.
Dosage: Dissolve 5 pellets under the tongue every 2 to 4 hours, as required.

+ **Arsenicum 6C**
Properties: For burning nasal discharge which irritates the nostrils and upper lip.
Dosage: Dissolve 5 pellets under the tongue every 2 to 4 hours, as required.

+ **Bryonia 6C**
Properties: For frequent sneezing, congestions, dull pain over the forehead, mouth and dry throat.
Dosage: Dissolve 5 pellets under the tongue every 2 to 4 hours, as required.

+ Ferrum phos. 6X

Properties: For feverishness, stuffiness and sneezing.

Dosage: Dissolve 5 pellets under the tongue every 1 to 2 hours, as required.

+ Natrum mur. 6X

Properties: For runny nose with chilliness and a general feeling of discomfort, cold sores.

Dosage: Dissolve 5 pellets under the tongue every 1 to 2 hours, as required.

+ Pulsatilla 6C

Properties: For nasal congestion, dry mouth.

Dosage: Dissolve 5 pellets under the tongue every 2 to 4 hours, as required.

+ Rhus tox. 6C

Properties: For chills, aches, restlessness, fever, dry cough.

Dosage: Dissolve 5 pellets under the tongue every 2 to 4 hours, as required.

+ Diet

It is important at the first sign of a cold, to stop eating dairy products and foods made with flour. These are considered mucous-forming foods. Also refrain from eating sugared foods, as they have a detrimental effect on the immune system.

+ Green tea

Properties: Immune booster and high antioxidant. Inhibits influenza. Very high in zinc for reducing sore throat pain.

Dosage: Mix 1 teaspoon of tea in small teapot. Steep for at least 1 minute. Strain and drink several times per day.

CUTS/WOUNDS

Quick Reference:

Nutritional Care:
Vitamin C
Vitamin E
Zinc

Herbal:
Aged Garlic Extract
Calendula
Catnip
Cayenne
Combination spray
Nature's Antiseptic
Rhododendron caucasicum
Tee Tree Oil

Homeopathic:
Arnica 6C or 30C
Hypericum 6C or 30C
Ledum 30C

Home Remedies:
First Aid flower remedy
Hydrogen Peroxide

Treatment Details:

Please refer to the American Red Cross technique for cleaning and bandaging wounds. Clean the wound with fresh water. Once you are satisfied the wound is clean, you can follow the listed recommendations. If profuse bleeding occurs, contact a health practitioner immediately.

Nutritional Care	*Cuts/Wounds*

+ Vitamin C
Properties: May help prevent infection and speed wound healing.
Dosage: 1,000 mg. from mixed mineral ascorbates 3 to 4 times per day, as required.

+ Vitamin E
Properties: May speed healing and prevent scar tissue from forming.
External application: Puncture a natural vitamin E capsule, and apply twice daily after the wound has closed up.

+ Zinc (for persons over 14 years of age)
Properties: May speed wound healing
Dosage: 50 mg of elemental zinc from amino acid chelate taken with a meal for 1 week, or until wound has completely healed.

+ Aged Garlic Extract

Properties: For open wounds to prevent infection.

External application: Use aged garlic extract liquid, and dribble into wound and bandage. Repeat each day until wound starts to close.

+ Calendula oil or cream

Properties: Available in an oil or cream, calendula should be applied externally, <u>after a wound has closed</u> and risk of infection is past,7 to speed healing and reduce infection.

External application:: Apply 3-4 times per day

+ Catnip

Properties: Catnip can be used where antiseptics and clean water are unavailable. Applied externally, it can be a temporary antiseptic and antiobiotic.

External application: Tear off several catnip leaves from the plant, crush and wet them with saliva. Apply crushed leaves to your cut, keeping them moist.

+Cayenne pepper
Properties: May stop bleeding. For minor bleeding only.
Dosage: Wash wound well, then sprinkle cayenne directly on cut. May cause stinging sensation.

+Combination spray (horsetail, chamomile, comfrey, burdock, green nettles, sage, rosemary,)
Properties: Use to accelerate healing and keep wound clean.
External application: Spray as needed on open or closed wound.

+Nature's Antiseptic (artemesia tridentata, chaparral, goldenseal, myrrh gum, echinacea, pau d'arco, yerba mansa, cayenne, oregano, horehound)
Properties: For both internal and external infections, including Staph, open sores, sore throat, stomach virus. A natural germicide.
Dosage: For tinctures, as listed on each specific bottle, 4 times per day. Small children should receive ¼ to ½ the suggested amount.

+Rhododendron caucasicum
Properties: Powerful antioxidant. Prevents infection. Beneficial healing properties.
Dosage: 3 capsules per day.

+ Tea Tree oil

Properties: Beneficial healing properties, antiseptic.

External application: Apply undiluted 1 to 2 drops or more, according to size of cut, each time wound is washed. May burn if used on sensitive areas, but pain can be minimized if diluted with olive oil.

Homeopathic remedies may be negated by strong stimulants such as black tea, excessive amounts of chocolate, camphor, coffee, mint, and strong odors such as garlic.

Choose from the following remedies, depending on the type of injury you are suffering from. Strength of remedy (12C, 6X) will be indicated on supplement.

+ Arnica 6C or 30C
Properties: Helps reduce pain.
Dosages: Dissolve 5 pellets under tongue immediately after injury. Repeat 1 to 3 times per day for 2 days.

+ Hypericum 6C or 30C
Properties: Cuts in fingertips, or if cut is infected or deep and there is shooting pain.
Dosages: Dissolve 5 pellets under the tongue 1 to 3 times daily, as required.

+ Ledum 30C
Properties: For puncture wounds inflicted by a sharp instrument, or after injection when area is sore. Particularly useful when extremities are cold.
Dosage: Dissolve 5 pellets under the tongue 1 to 3 times daily, as required.

+ **First Aid Flower Remedy** (cherry plum, clematis, impatiens, rock rose, and Star of Bethlehem)

Properties: Gives relief and healing during and following emergencies, accidents, shock, injury, insect and animal bites or any trauma or terror.

Dosage: 3 drops orally under the tongue in 5-10 minute intervals, as needed.

+ **Hydrogen peroxide (3 %)**

Properties: May be used to disinfect.

External application: Pour into wound, let foam, then repeat and pat dry with clean gauze or cotton. May be used to cleanse wound before each application of oils or cream listed above.

DIARRHEA

Quick Reference:

Nutritional Care:
Digestive Enzymes
Electrolyte trace minerals
Probiotics

Herbal:
Bowel tonic
Ginger
Golden Seal

Homeopathic:
Aconite 12C
Arsenicum 6C
Kali Mur 6X
Nitric acid 30C
Nux Vomica 12C
Pulsatilla 6C

Home Remedies:
Water
Activated Charcoal

Treatment Details:

Warning: Diarrhea can cause severe dehydration, and may be life-threatening, especially to infants, children and the elderly. Also review any remedy with a pediatrician for children prior to utilization.

Nutritional Care	*Diarrhea*

+ Digestive Enzymes
Properties: Enzymes assist with digestion of food and normalization of the digestive tract. It is recommended to take plant enzymes that work throughout the entire digestive tract.
Dosage: Generally 2-3 capsules with meals. Follow directions on bottles of specific supplement.

+ Electrolyte Trace Minerals
Properties: Provides needed electrolytes that are lost due to diarrhea and removal of water from the system.
Dosage: (Liquid electrolyte solutions) Take 1 tsp. in 8 oz. water, 3 times per day.

+ **Probiotics**

These are friendly intestinal bacteria which aid digestion, nutrient assimilation and toxin elimination; examples: L. acidophilus.

Properties: Replaces friendly bacteria lost as result of diarrhea.

Dosage: Use according to directions on label.

+ **Bowel tonic** (fennel, cascara segrada, senna pods, rhubarb root, buckthorn, black walnut, slippery elm, licorice, oregon grape, ginger, cayenne)

Properties: Supplies nutrients to the lower bowel, reducing causes of diarrhea.

Dosage: For tinctures, as listed on each specific bottle, 4 times per day. Small children should receive ¼ to ½ the suggested amount.

+ **Ginger**

Properties: To reduce bouts of diarrhea.

Dosage: Make a tea with ginger, and drink it several hours apart.

Note: If the diarrhea continues for more than 2 days, the cause may be viral, and you may switch to golden seal.

+ **Goldenseal**

Properties: Traditionally used as an antibacterial and antibiotic. May be beneficial when diarrhea is accompanied by fever, which may indicate bacterial infection.

Dosage: 2-4 capsules or 40-50 drops of liquid extract three times daily for up to 14 days.

Note: Decrease dosage if diarrhea becomes worse.

Homeopathic remedies may be negated by strong stimulants such as black tea, excessive amounts of chocolate, camphor, coffee, mint, and strong odors such as garlic.

Choose from the following remedies, depending on the type of diarrhea you are suffering from. Strength of remedy (12C, 6X) will be indicated on supplement.

+ Aconite 12C

Properties: Diarrhea brought on by exposure to cold temperatures, or as the result of fright.

Dosage: 5 pellets dissolved under the tongue every 1-2 hours 3-4 times per day, as required. For infants, crush pellets and dissolve in 4-oz water. Administer 1 tsp. every 2 to 4 hours, as required.

+ Arsenicum 6C

Properties: Diarrhea from food poisoning or stomach flu.

Dosage: 5 pellets dissolved under the tongue every 1-2 hours 3-4 times per day, as required. For infants, crush pellets and dissolve in 4-oz water. Administer 1 tsp. every 1 to 3 hours, as required.

+ Kali Mur 6X

Properties: For diarrhea from fatty or rich foods.

Dosage: Dissolve 5 pellets under the tongue 3 to 6 times daily, as required. For infants, crush pellets and dissolve in 4-oz water. Administer 1 tsp. every 1 to 3 hours, as required.

+ Nitric acid 30C

Properties: Diarrhea from antibiotic use.

Dosage: Dissolve 5 pellets under the tongue every 2 hours until relief is obtained. For infants, crush pellets and dissolve in 4 oz water. Administer 1 tsp. every 2- 4 hours, as required.

+ Nux Vomica 12C

Properties: Diarrhea from Dietary, alcohol and drug indiscretion.

Dosage: Dissolve 5 pellets under the tongue 2 to 4 times daily, as required. For infants, crush pellets and dissolve in 4-oz water. Administer 1 tsp. every 2 to 4 hours. as required.

+ Pulsatilla 6C

Properties: Diarrhea from eating too much fruit, rich or greasy foods, from cold food or drinks.

Dosage: Dissolve 5 pellets under the tongue 2 to 4 times daily, as required. For infants, crush pellets and dissolve in 4-oz water. Administer 1 tsp. every 2 to 4 hours, as required.

+ **Water**

Drink generous amounts of liquids, including purified water, herbal teas, soups, and diluted vegetable juices. Fluids help prevent dehydration, and replace lost electrolytes and vitamins.

Note: Low-sugar fluid-replacement drinks that include electrolytes are very beneficial.

+ **Activated charcoal**

Properties: Absorbs diarrhea-producing toxins in the bowel.

Dosage: 1 tsp. dissolved in 8-oz. water, or 2 capsules activated charcoal every 3 hours for up to 5 days, then reduce dosage as required.

Charcoal Warning: Long term use of charcoal may impair nutrient absorption from the digestive system.

HEADACHE

Quick Reference:

Nutritional Care:
Calcium
Magnesium
Vitamin B-complex

Herbal:
Chaste Tree Berry
Feverfew
Pain combination
Peppermint oil
Valerian root
White Willow

Homeopathic:
Aconite 12C
Arnica 12C
Belladonna 12C
Ferrum Phos. 6X
Nat Mur. 6X
Nux Vomica 12C

Home Remedies:
Flower remedy
Water plus electrolytes

Treatment Details:

Recommendations below are for general head-aches. Prolonged or severe symptoms are a sign that proper medical attention should be sought.

Nutritional Care	*Headache*

+ Calcium
Properties: Essential for the relaxation of the nervous system. Considered a "lullaby" mineral.
Dosage: 500 to 1,000 mg daily dose of elemental calcium from amino acid chelate in divided doses, with meals and at bedtime. Should be taken simultaneously with magnesium.
Note: If headaches occur at consistent times, take two hours before expected time.

+ Magnesium
Properties: Relaxes the nervous system.
Dosage: 500 to 1,000 mg daily in divided doses, with meals and at bedtime. Use elemental magnesium made from amino acid chelate. Should be taken simultaneously with calcium.
Note: If headaches occur at consistent times, take two hours before expected time of onset. High doses may cause loose stools.

+ Vitamin B-complex

Properties: For headache prevention: helps support the nervous system.

Dosage: 50 mg balanced B-complex capsule; use daily.

+ **Chaste Tree berries**
Properties: For headaches made worse by hormonal imbalance.
Dosage: As a preventive: 2 capsules or 1 teaspoon of liquid extract upon awakening, for at least 90 days.

+ **Feverfew**
Properties: Traditionally used for pain relief in ways similar to aspirin, but without aspirin's stomach-irritant property. Particularly beneficial for migraines, and may be used long term as a method of prevention.
Dosage: 1 to 2 capsules twice daily as required.
Note: Take for a minimum of 90 days, for preventive measures.

+ **Pain combination** (black willow, cramp bark, valerian, wild lettuce, scullcap,. wintergreen, dillweed, thyme, wild lettuce, cayenne)
Properties: Supplies nutrients to the body for eliminating the causes of headaches.
Dosage: Tinctures: As listed on each specific bottle, 4 times per day. Small children should receive ¼ to ½ the suggested amount.

+ Peppermint oil

Properties: Headaches from eyestrain or stress.
External applications: Use an essential oil of peppermint and dab a drop on each temple, as well as one on the nape of the neck. Make a tea of peppermint leaves; moisten a washcloth with the tea and apply to your forehead.
Internal dosage: Drink tea made from peppermint leaves.

+ Valerian root

Properties: Valerian calms nerves and acts as a sedative.
Dosage: 2 capsules or 30 to 60 drops of liquid extract in 4 oz. water; drink 2 to 3 times per day.

+ White willow

Conditions: Commonly know as herbal aspirin, it will work for anything you normally use aspirin for, such as headache, pain, fever and inflammation.
Dosage: 30 drops of liquid extract in 4 oz. water, 2-3 times per day.

Homeopathic remedies may be negated by strong stimulants such as black tea, excessive amounts of chocolate, camphor, coffee, mint, and strong odors such as garlic.

Choose from the following remedies, depending on the type of headache you are suffering from. Strength of remedy (12C, 6X) will be indicated on supplement.

+ Aconite 12C
Properties: Take for symptoms: sudden, violent headaches that feel as if the skull will burst out through the forehead..
Dosage: 5 pellets under the tongue, every hour until pain begins to subside.

+ Arnica 12C
Properties: Take for headaches caused by a blow to the head, or other form of head trauma.
Dosage: 5 pellets under the tongue, every hour until pain begins to subside.

+ Belladonna 12C
Properties: Take for symptoms: throbbing headaches with violent shooting pains.
Dosage: 5 pellets under the tongue, every hour until pain begins to subside.

+ Ferrum Phos. 6X

Properties: Use for headache resulting from either extreme cold, or the heat of the sun.

Dosage: 5 pellets under the tongue every 15 minutes, until pain begins to subside.

+ Nat Mur. 6X

Properties: Take for symptoms: dull, heavy headache with drowsiness and disturbed sleep that is made worse by thinking, reading, excessive eye movement, and excessive exposure to strong sunlight.

Dosage: 5 pellets under the tongue every 30 minutes, until pain begins to subside.

+ Nux Vomica 12C

Properties: Take for symptoms: a splitting headache that is often accompanied by nausea and vomiting.

Dosage: 5 pellets under the tongue every hour, until pain begins to subside.

+ **Flower remedy** (aspen, dandelion, impatiens, lotus, sweet chestnut, vervain, chamomile, white chestnut)

Properties: To help release mental strain and pressure. Relaxes tense muscles, calms and strengthens the nervous system, and eases tension headaches and pain.

Dosage: 3 drops orally under the tongue, in water or juice, as often as necessary. For chronic conditions: take dosage 4 times per day.

+ **Water plus electrolytes**

Properties: Many headaches originate because of dehydration from long exposure to sun or dry climates. Useful for headaches that occur after strenuous exercise with profuse sweating.

Dosage: 1 tsp. of liquid electrolyte supplement in 8 oz. water every 15 minutes, for at least an hour.

INDIGESTION

Quick Reference:

Nutritional Care:
Calcium
Digestive Enzymes
Magnesium
Probiotics

Herbal:
Chamomile
Indigestion combination
Ginger root
Peppermint leaf

Homeopathic:
Arsenicum album 12C
Carbo vegetabalis 6C
Nat Mur. 6X
Nux Vomica 12C
Pulsatilla 6C

Home Remedies:
Apple Cider Vinegar

Treatment Details:

Treatments indicated are for occasional indigestion, or prevention of symptoms. Persons with chronic conditions should seek proper medical attention.

| *Nutritional Care* | *Indigestion* |

+ Calcium
Properties: Essential for the relaxation of the nervous system. Considered a "lullaby" mineral.
Dosage: 500 to 1,000 mg daily of elemental calcium from amino acid chelate in divided doses, with meals and at bedtime. Should be taken with magnesium.

+ Digestive Enzymes
Properties: Enzymes assist with digestion of food and normalization of the digestive juices. It is recommended to take plant enzymes that work throughout the entire digestive tract.
Dosage: Generally 2-3 capsules with meals, or during upset. Follow directions on bottles of specific supplement.

+ Magnesium

Properties: Essential for the relaxation of the nervous system.

Dosage: 500 to 1,000 mg daily in divided doses with meals and at bedtime of elemental, magnesium from amino acid chelate. Should be taken in conjunction with calcium

+ Probiotics

Properties: Probiotics are friendly intestinal bacteria that aid digestion, nutrient assimilation and toxin elimination such as L. acidophilus.

Dosage: according to directions on label.

Avialable in powder or capsule form.

+ **Chamomile flowers**
Properties: May be beneficial for stress-related indigestion. Antispasmodic and soothing to the nerves.
Dosage: 6 oz. of tea three times daily, between meals. Prepare as follows: Place 1 heaping teaspoon of the herb in a non-aluminum cooking pot (preferably glass). Pour 8 oz boiling pure water over herbs. Cover, and let steep for 20 minutes. Strain and drink while still warm.

+ **Indigestion combination** (fennel, chamomile, wild yam, catnip, liverwort, papaya, clovers, ginger, star anise, peppermint, dillweed, cayenne)
Properties: Effective for easing the effects of overeating, stomach and intestinal gas. It strongly helps in the elimination of uric acid.
Dosage: Tinctures: As listed on each specific bottle, 4 times per day. Small children should receive ¼ to ½ the suggested amount.

+ **Ginger root**
Properties: May aid with digestion and reduce gas and bloating.
Dosage: 2 capsules or 4 oz. of dried ginger root tea before each meal

+ **Peppermint leaf**

Propertiess: May aid in digestion, and soothe the stomach. Peppermint candy can be used if necessary, but the sugar may aggravate the indigestion.

Dosage: Take one cup of peppermint tea after each meal.

Homeopathic remedies may be negated by strong stimulants such as black tea, excessive amounts of chocolate, camphor, coffee, mint, and strong odors such as garlic.

Choose from the following remedies, depending on the type of indigestion you are suffering from. Strength of remedy (12C, 6X) will be indicated on supplement.

+ Arsenicum Album 12C
Properties: For a burning pain in the stomach that occurs soon after eating and is relieved by warm drinks.
Dosage: 5 pellets under the tongue, hourly until symptom subsides.

+ Carbo Vegetabalis 6C
Properties: For pain and tenderness in the pit of the stomach that occurs within 30 minutes after eating.
Dosage: 5 pellets under the tongue, hourly until symptom subsides.

+ Nat Mur. 6X
Properties: Use for heartburn after eating, during pregnancy.
Dosage: 5 pellets under the tongue, every 30 minutes until symptom subsides.

+ Nux Vomica 12C

Properties: Take for symptoms: heartburn and gas from over-indulgence in coffee, tobacco and alcohol.

Dosage: 5 pellets under the tongue, hourly until symptoms diminish.

+ Pulsatilla 6C

Properties: Take for symptoms: bloating with a sensation of having eaten too much, and of having to loosen clothing.

Dosage: 5 pellets under the tongue, hourly until symptom subsides.

+ Unfiltered apple cider vinegar

Properties: For all indigestion. Increases salivary flow and the secretion of digestive fluids in the stomach.

Dosage: 2 drops of apple cider vinegar in 1 tablespoon pure water, 5 minutes before eating. Hold in the mouth for 15 seconds, then swallow.

Quick Reference:

Nutritional Care:
Calcium/magnesium
Melatonin
Vitamin B complex
Vitamin B_3

Herbal:
Chamomile tea
Kava kava
Valerian

Homeopathic:
Chamomilla 6X
Kali phos, 6X
Nux vomica 12C

Treatment Details:

Treatments indicated are for occasional problems with insomnia, or prevention of symptoms. Persons with chronic conditions should seek proper medical attention.

Nutritional Care	Insomnia

+ Calcium/Magnesium
Properties: Considered a "lullaby" mineral. Essential for relaxation of the nervous system.
Dosage: 1,000 mg of elemental calcium and magnesium combination at bedtime.

+ Melatonin
Properties: A natural hormone produced in the brain to help with sleep, and reset your internal clock.
Dosage: 3 mg ½ hour before bedtime.

+ Vitamin B complex
Properties: Helps the body cope with stress.
Dosage: 50 mg 1 to 2 times daily, with meals.

+ Vitamin B$_3$ (Niacinamide)
Properties: For symptoms: you fall asleep easily, but cannot return to sleep after waking.
Dosage: 1,000 mg at bedtime
Note: This is niacinamide, NOT niacin.

+ Chamomile tea

Properties: Soothing to the nerves. Excellent for difficult children, who are perpetually dissatisfied.

Dosage: 4 to 8 oz. of tea ½ hour before bedtime.

+ Kava kava

Properties: Has significant relaxant properties. May benefit an overactive mind.

Dosage: 2 capsules of a standardized extract, or 30 drops of liquid extract in 4 oz. of water, ½ hour before bedtime.

+ Valerian root

Properties: Valerian is best suited for those individuals who are awakened by the slightest noise, and are prone to fears at night.

Dosage: 2 capsules, or 30 to 60 drops of liquid extract in 4 oz. of water ½ hour before bedtime, or capsules as directed on the bottle.

Homeopathic remedies may be negated by strong stimulants such as black tea, excessive amounts of chocolate, camphor, coffee, mint and strong odors such as garlic.

Choose from the following remedies, depending on the type of insomnia you are suffering from. Strength of remedy (12C, 6X) will be indicated on supplement.

+ Chamomilla 6X
Properties: For difficulty falling asleep due to irritability or pain.
Dosage: 5 pellets under the tongue 30 minutes before bedtime; hourly thereafter as required.

+ Kali phos, 6X
Properties: For people who awaken with night terrors, and have difficulty falling asleep again.
Dosage: 5 pellets under the tongue 30 minutes before bedtime; hourly thereafter as required.

+ Nux vomica 12C
Properties: For sleeplessness due to use of alcohol, coffee, tea, tobacco, prescription medications or rich foods.
Dosage: 5 pellets under the tongue 1 to 2 times daily, as required.

NAUSEA/MOTION SICKNESS

Quick Reference:

Nutritional Care:
Manganese
Vitamin B_6
Zinc

Herbal:
Combination remedy
Herbal Blend tea
Ginger root
Goldenseal
Peppermint

Homeopathic:
Cocculus 6C
Ferrum phos. 6X
Ipecac 6C
Nux Vomica 12C
Tabacum 12C

Home Remedies:
Flower remedies
Ginger cookies
Soda crackers

Treatment Details:

Various remedies listed below consider the type of condition in parenthesis. For nausea associated with pregnancy, women should speak to their OBGYN or health-care practitioner before taking any new supplements.

Nutritional Care	*Nausea/Motion sickness*

+ Manganese

Properties: Manganese is necessary as a precursor for SOD, which is the major antioxidant in the human body. Clinical evidence shows that manganese is helpful in cases of nausea from pregnancy and motion sickness.

Dosage: 5 to 10 mg (aspartate or citrate) 1 to 3 times daily, with meals.

+ Vitamin B_6
(Pregnancy)

Properties: For morning sickness

Dosage: 25 to 50 mg daily with breakfast and dinner.

Notes: 1) Always use B_6 in conjunction with a complete B-complex formula, as high doses of one of the B-Vitamins may imbalance other vitamins in the body. 2) Reduce dosage as frequency and intensity of morning sickness diminishes. 3) After delivery, dosage of Vitamin B_6 should be reduced to no more than 25 mg. daily, as high doses of this vitamin may inhibit the flow of breast milk.

+ Zinc
(Pregnancy)
Properties: Used for morning sickness in pregnant women over 14 years of age. Zinc is a Vitamin B_6 synergist, and may also help prevent post-partum depression.

Dosage: 25 mg of elemental zinc from amino acid chelate, taken with breakfast and dinner.

+Combination Remedy (ginger, cassia, clove bud, hyssop, black caraway seed, nutmeg, peppermint, red poppy flower)
(General)
Properties: Reduces symptoms of motion sickness.
Dosage: Take for 5 days prior to travel. Tinctures: 10 drops 4 times per day. Small children should receive ¼ to ½ the suggested amount.

+ Herbal Blend tea
(General)
Cloves, Ginger or Cinnamon mixed into Chamomile tea (Matricaria chamomilla) or Peppermint tea.
Prepare as follows: Add a pinch of either powdered cloves, ginger or cinnamon to 6 oz. of warm chamomile or peppermint tea, to help allay morning sickness or other forms of nausea.

+ Ginger root
(General)
Properties: Excellent for most cases of nausea.
Notes: Generally safe and effective for pregnancy; however, always speak to your healthcare practitioner before adding any new herb.

Dosage: 2 500 mg. capsules 3-times daily, or 6 to 8 oz. of dried ginger root tea, 3 times daily.
(Travel)
Properties: For prevention of motion sickness. Additional capsules may be used every four to five hours during travel, as needed.
Dosage: Two 500 mg capsules, 30 to 60 minutes before trip begins.

+ Goldenseal root
(Pregnancy)
Properties: May help to ameliorate chronic morning sickness.
Dosage: 1 capsule after breakfast and dinner.

+ Peppermint
Properties: May help to soothe the stomach. Peppermint is most beneficial for nausea if taken after the stomach has emptied. Do not take peppermint candies that contain sugar, as the sweetener has an adverse affect on the stomach.
Dosage: 8 oz. of warm tea, 90 minutes after meals.

Homeopathic remedies may be negated by strong stimu-lants such as black tea, excessive amounts of chocolate, camphor, coffee, mint, and strong odors such as garlic.

Choose from the following remedies, depending on the type of nausea you are suffering from. Strength of remedy (12C, 6X) will be indicated on supplement.

+ Cocculus 6C
(Travel)
Properties: A primary remedy for travel sickness.
Dosage: 5 pellets under the tongue, hourly as required until symptoms subside.

+ Ferrum Phos. 6X
(Pregnancy)
Properties: Take for symptoms: vomiting dur-ing pregnancy, when food is regurgitated undi-gested.
Dosage: 5 pellets taken under the tongue 3 to 4 times daily upon arising, and 30 minutes before meals.

+ Ipecac 6C
(General & Pregnancy)
Properties: Take for symptoms: persistent nausea and vomiting, when the nausea is not relieved by the vomiting. Often associated with the ingestion of rich, difficult-to-digest foods. May also prove beneficial for morning sickness.
Dosage: 5 pellets under the tongue, hourly as required, until symptoms subside.

+ Nux Vomica 12C
(General & Pregnancy)
Properties: Take for symptoms: often related to overindulgence in alcohol or food, or mental overwork. May be specific for cases of morning sickness when morning nausea is typically accompanied by a sour taste in the mouth upon awakening.
Dosage: 5 pellets under the tongue, hourly as required until symptoms subside.

+ Tabacum 12C
(Travel)
Properties: For travel sickness when there is dizziness and nausea accompanied by coldness, faintness, sweating and a sinking feeling in the stomach.
Dosage: 5 pellets under the tongue, hourly as required until symptoms subside.

+ **Flower remedy** (aspen, blackberry, cherry plum, garlic, mimulus, red chestnut, rock rose.)
Properties: A combination that is used for fear and anxiety (such as fear of flying) that can manifest in nausea, sweats or light-headedness.
Dosage: 3 to 10 drops at onset of symptoms, then 3 drops every 5-10 minutes as needed, until anxiety subsides.

+ **Ginger cookies**
If you don't happen to have access to ginger powder, buy a bag of ginger cookies. Especially good to have along on car or boat trips.

+ **Soda crackers**
Sometimes, eating a carbohydrate, such as soda crackers or bread, can reduce the nausea.

SORE THROAT

Quick Reference:

Nutritional Care:
Vitamin A
Vitamin C
Zinc

Herbal:
Aged garlic extract
Echinacea
Goldenseal

Homeopathic:
Aconite 6C
Belladonna 6C
Calcarea phos. 6X
Ferrum phos. 6X
Kali mur. 6X

Home Remedies:
Cayenne-Apple Cider Vinegar
Green tea
Heating compress

Treatment Details:

| *Nutritional Care* | *Sore Throat* |

+ **Vitamin A** (natural, from fish liver oil)
Properties: Vitamin A is essential for the maintenance of mucous membranes, including those of the throat.
Dosage: 25,000 IU to 50,000 IU per day, taken with meals, for one week only.
Note: Consult a physician before using higher doses of Vitamin A. <u>Avoid use if pregnant</u>. Discontinue use if it produces nausea, dry skin, sore lips, blurred vision or other signs of Vitamin A excess.

+ **Vitamin C**
Properties: May stimulate immune function and aid in the prevention or treatment of infection.
Dosage: 1,000 mg. 4 to 6 times daily, or to normal bowel tolerance--the point at which tissue saturation with Vitamin C has been reached, and the body will not absorb any more vitamin C from the digestive tract. The point of normal bowel tolerance of vitamin C is ascertained by taking 1,000 mg of vitamin C per hour until characteristic symptoms, including rumbling flatus and looser stool, occur. Then reduce dosage to 1,000 mg 4 to 6 times daily, as required.

+ Zinc (if over 14 years of age)

Properties: Zinc plays an important role in immune function, and greater amounts are required during acute or chronic infection.

Dosage: Zinc lozenges containing 23 mg of elemental zinc, dissolved in the mouth every two hours during waking hours. Limit intake of zinc at this high dosage level to no more than 7 to 10 days.

+ Aged Garlic extract capsules
Properties: Powerful antiviral and antibacterial
Dosage: 1 to 2 capsules of aged garlic extract per meal. Fresh, raw garlic can be used. Garlic has a greater effect when taken with echinacea.
Note: Raw parsley taken with raw garlic will help prevent "garlic breath" and enhance garlic's blood-cleansing effects.

+ Echinacea
Properties: Traditionally used to stimulate the immune system and help fight infections.
Dosage: 2 to 4 capsules, or 50 drops of liquid extract every two hours, until throat symptoms subside. Echinacea has a noteworthy affinity with garlic, and so these two can be used to greater effect when taken in combination.

+ Goldenseal
Properties: Traditionally used as a cleanser of mucous membranes and an antibacterial which may have specificity for streptococcal infection.
Dosage: Gargle, then swallow 40 to 50 drops of liquid extract in 4oz of warm water, every three hours, until throat symptoms subside.

Homeopathic remedies may be negated by strong stimulants such as black tea, excessive amounts of chocolate, camphor, coffee, mint and strong odors such as garlic.

Choose from the following remedies, depending on the type of sore throat you are suffering from. Strength of remedy (12C, 6X) will be indicated on supplement.

+ Aconite 6C

Properties: For first stage of sore throat, perhaps accompanied by fever, which comes on suddenly and intensely after exposure to cold air or dry, cold wind.

Dosage: 5 pellets under the tongue, every 2 to 4 hours, as required.

+ Belladonna 6C

Properties: Take for symptoms: acute tonsillitis; throat that is very dry, with intense burning sensation; tonsils and tongue are bright red; there is tickling of the larynx.

Dosage: 5 pellets under the tongue, every 1 to 4 hours, as required.

+ Calcarea phos. 6X

Properties: Take for symptoms: sore, aching throat with much pain upon swallowing. The sore throat may be caused by excessive speaking or lecturing.

Dosage: 5 pellets under the tongue, every 3 to 4 hours, as required.

+ Ferrum phos. 6X

Properties: Take for symptoms: dry, red and inflamed throat, with throbbing pain and burning sensation.

Dosage: 5 pellets under the tongue, every 1 to 4 hours, as required. Most effective if taken at the onset of the sore throat.

+ Kali mur. 6X

Properties: Take for symptoms: swelling of glands or enlargement of tonsils.

Dosage: 5 pellets under the tongue, every 2 to 4 hours, alternating with Ferrum phos., as required.

+ Cayenne-Apple Cider Vinegar gargle

Properties: May help stimulate local circulatory and immunological activity.

Dosage: Mix together: 1 teaspoon cayenne powder, 8 oz. sage (salvia officinalis) tea prepared by infusion (*see Appendix B*), 2 tablespoons unfiltered apple cider vinegar, 2 tablespoons sea salt and 2 tablespoons raw honey. Steep sage infusion mixed with cayenne for 15 minutes, then mix in the remaining ingredients. Gargle with a mouthful of this blend, 4 to 8 times daily. After spitting out the gargle, take orally, and swallow 1 to 2 tablespoons of this same blend.

+ Green tea

Properties: Immune booster and high antioxidant. Inhibits influenza. Very high in zinc for reducing sore throat pain.

Dosage: Mix 1 teaspoon of tea in small teapot. Steep for at least 1 minute. Strain and drink several times per day.

+ Heating compress

Properties: May help to soothe the throat area and stimulate the immune system.

External application: Place a cold, damp cloth (wring it out) on the throat, and wrap the entire neck area with a dry towel. Leave this on your throat for an hour (towel should feel warm).

SPRAINS

Quick Reference:

Nutritional Care:
Bioflavonoids
Bromelain
Proteolytic Enzymes
Velvet antler

Herbal:
Cayenne
Comfrey
Pain combination
Rhododendron caucasicum
White willow bark

Homeopathic:
Arnica oil or gel
Bryonia 6C
Ferrum Phos. 6X
Magnesia Phos. 6X
Rhus. Tox 6C

Home Remedies:
Cabbage compress
First Aid Flower Remedy
Green Tea
Hot/Cold compress
Ice

Treatment Details:

Remedies suggested are to alleviate immediate pain, and also to be taken as a preventive measure against future trauma.

Nutritional Care	*Sprain*

+ Bioflavonoids (full potency bioflavonoids)
Properties: May help limit ruptures in capillaries and connective tissues.
Dosage: 500 mg, 2 to 3 times daily.

+ Bromelain
Properties: Enzyme derived from pineapple. Reduces inflammation and speeds healing.
Dosage: Two 5000 mcg (measure of bromelain activity) capsules, three times daily between meals.

+ Proteolytic Enzyme Formula
Properties: Can decrease inflammation and speed healing of tissues if taken between meals. If taken with meals, the enzymes are used up in the digestive process.
Dosage: 3 or more capsules, three times daily between meals.
Note: Avoid if there are stomach or duodenal ulcers. Proteolytic enzymes may aggravate ulcers and induce bleeding.

+ Velvet Antler

Properties: Natural anti-inflammatory and anti-arthritic substance from antlers harvested humanely from elk. Contains collagen, condroiton sulfate and N-Acetyl-Glucosamine, all of which have been associated with accelerated wound healing.

Dosage: As per instructions on the supplement bottle. Normal dosage is 1-3 capsules per day.

+ Cayenne

Properties: Facilitates heat application.

External application: Make a cayenne liniment by combining 1 oz. of powdered cayenne in a quart-sized dark bottle filled with vodka or vinegar. Let stand in a cool place for 8-10 days, shaking it vigorously. Apply to affected area. The effects last 2-6 hours.

Note: For persons with sensitive or fair skin, test the liniment in a small a first, as it can cause blistering. Also avoid use if pregnant.

+ Comfrey

Properties: To reduce swelling and potential inflammation.

Dosage: As a tea, use only the leaf. Drink 1-4 cups per day, for a maximum of 14 days.

External application: Combine 2-3 tablespoons of dried powdered root with just enough boiling water to form a thick paste. Add a teaspoon of honey for extra drawing action. Mold with your hands into a ¼" thick slab, and place on affected area. Cover with gauze and leave in place for 4-8 hours, preferably elevating the affected area.

Caution: <u>Do not drink comfrey tea if you have a history of liver damage or liver cancer.</u>

+ Pain combination (black willow, cramp bark, valerian, wild lettuce, scullcap,. wintergreen, dillweed, thyme, wild lettuce, cayenne)

Properties: Supplies nutrients to the body for eliminating the causes of headaches.

Dosage: Tinctures: As listed on each specific bottle, 4 times per day. Small children should receive ¼ to ½ the suggested amount.

+ Rhododendron caucasicum

Properties; One of the most powerful antioxidants in the world. Helps to prevent inflammation, and is very beneficial for its healing properties for arthritis.

Dosage: 3 capsules per day.

+ White willow bark capsules

Properties: This herb has been used to relieve pain

Dosage: 2,000 mg. 2 to 3 times daily with meals, or 4 oz. of tea 2 to 3 times daily between meals.

Homeopathic remedies may be negated by strong stimulants such as black tea, excessive amounts of chocolate, camphor, coffee, mint, and strong odors such as garlic.

Choose from the following remedies, depending on the type of symptom you are suffering from. Strength of remedy (12C, 6X) will be indicated on supplement.

+ Arnica oil or gel
Properties: May help reduce swelling and speed healing. For best results, use immediately after injury.
External Application: Use externally by rubbing small amount into affected area 3 to 4 times daily, and after alternate hot and cold compress applications.
Note: **Toxic when taken internally**. Avoid mouth, eyes and any open cuts.

+ Bryonia 6C
Properties: Take for symptoms: a joint that is painful and distended with fluid, aggravated by the least amount of motion, and worse with continued motion.
Dosage: 5 pellets under the tongue, 3 to 4 times daily.

+ Ferrum Phos. 6X

Properties: First-aid remedy for sprains, given immediately after the occurrence of the injury. Helps alleviate pain and congestion.

External application: Crush tablets, dissolve in a little water and apply externally every 15 minutes for 3 hours, then hourly for 4 hours. Decrease to 2 to 4 times per day (in accordance with the severity of the injury) for the next 2 days.

+ Magnesia Phos. 6X

Properties: Tale for symptoms: spasmodic, vivid, shooting, burning or stitching pains that are sensitive to touch, and are better with warm applications.

Dosage: 5 Pellets dissolved under the tongue every 15 minutes (during acute pain), or 3 times per day, as required. Adjust dosage as symptoms subside.

+ Rhus Tox. 6C

Properties: <u>Primary homeopathic medicine for sprains</u> and muscle strains from overexertion. Joints are hot, swollen, stiff and painful. They are worse upon initial motion, but loosen up with continued motion. The pain is relieved by warmth, gentle rubbing and change of position.

Dosage: 5 pellets under the tongue, 3 to 4 times per day.

+ Cabbage compress
Properties: Swelling normally goes away in 3 consecutive treatments of this application. Also beneficial for water-on-the-knee.
External application: Prepare as follows: Take 3 or 4 leaves of green cabbage and cook until soft. Cool slightly and wrap around sprain before bedtime. Externally wrap plastic-wrap around cabbage, and then apply an ace-bandage. Undo the wrapping in the morning.

+ First Aid Flower Remedy
(cherry plum, clematis, impatiens, rock rose, and Star of Bethlehem)
Properties: Gives relief and healing during and following emergencies, accidents, shock, injury, insect and animal bites or any trauma or terror.
Dosage: 3 drops orally under the tongue in 5-10 minute intervals, as needed.

+ Green tea
Properties: Immune booster and high antioxidant. Anti-inflammatory agent.
Dosage: Mix 1 teaspoon of tea in small teapot. Steep for at least 1 minute. Strain and drink several times per day.

+ Alternate hot and cold compresses or soaks

Properties: Encourages vigorous blood circulation and reduces tissue swelling

External application: The alternate hot and cold soak is preferred for ankle, elbow or wrist. Begin 24 hours after the time of injury. Can use salt water for increased effectiveness. Dry the affected part, and bandage for support. Repeat 2 to 3 times daily, as required.

+ Ice

Properties: Reduce swelling

External application: Apply ice to the injured area immediately, to reduce inflammation and pain. Keep the ice pack in place for 5 minutes. Remove for 1-2 minutes and repeat, as needed.

Appendix

+ Internal Herbal Applications

Alcohol tinctures

Tinctures, also known as herbal extracts, are a concentrated form of herbal medicine. They are prepared by soaking the herb in alcohol to extract the herb's beneficial properties. In this form, herbs are extremely potent and are usually taken mixed in tea, water or juice. Caution should be taken when combining several tinctures, as this can cause high levels of alcohol to be ingested.

Glycerite tinctures

Glycerites are syrupy liquids that provide an alcohol-free alternative to tinctures. They are made with glycerin, not alcohol. This produces a sweet taste, but does not affect blood-sugar levels. Glycerites are generally diluted in water, tea or juice, because they can irritate the mouth if taken full strength. They are not as potent as tinctures, but they are often recommended for use by children and people wishing to avoid alcohol.

Supplements

Pills come in both tablet and capsule form. They are generally made from either dried herbs or liquid tinctures combined with a filler. The advantage of taking pills is that they are convenient, are alcohol free, and you do not taste the herb when swallowing. This can be a disadvantage with some herbs where the taste contributes to its effectiveness. Pills have a shorter shelf-life than tinctures and are less potent. Vegetarians should be careful to avoid gelatin capsules that are made from a meat derivative. To assure freshness, break open a capsule and make sure the smell, color, and taste are similar to that of the original herb.

Tea Infusion

Teas are one of the least expensive ways to take herbs. They can be prepared as hot infusions, cold infusions, or decoctions. Although tea bags are the most common form of infusion, loose herbs can often create a fresher and more powerful tea. Hot infusions are prepared by placing one tablespoon of herb in a non-aluminum cooking pot (preferably glass), and pouring two cups of pure boiling water over the herbs. Cover and let steep for 20 to 30 minutes; strain and drink while still warm. Cold infusions are made by soaking the herbs in cold water for about eight hours. This form is less frequently used. Decoctions are prepared by gently simmering the herbs for 15 to 30 minutes. This is usually done with roots and barks.

Caution: Never take herbs or any other supplements if you are pregnant, nursing, being treated for any other illness, or taking any other medications, without consulting your health-care practitioner. Always follow recommended doses. If you experience any side affects, discontinue use and notify your health care practitioner. Parents should not give any herbs to children without prior consultation with their pediatrician. Never discontinue any prescribed medication without consulting your health-care practitioner.

+External Herbal Applications

Compress

A compress is an easy way to use herbs externally. Take a clean cloth (cheese cloth or clean cotton), and soak it in warm (not hot), strong herbal tea, diluted tincture or glycerite, essential oil or aromatic water. Wring out and place the warm cloth over the affected area; cover the cloth with plastic or waxed paper and place a hot water bottle on top to keep warm.

Poultice

A poultice is a fresh plant that is crushed to form a paste. This paste can be applied directly to the affected area or mixed with hot water, hot apple cider vinegar or clay. It can also be placed between two thin layers of gauze and then placed onto affected area. Keep the poultice warm by placing over it, a hot water bottle.

Salve

A salve is a thick herbal oil that is used topically for skin problems. It is made by adding herbs to a thick vegetable oil, and may also be combined with beeswax to increase adherence to the skin.

Caution: Although poultices and compresses are made from natural substances, they have medicinal properties, and should be used with caution.

+Alternating hot and cold compresses

Constitutional Hydrotherapy

Traditionally used for conditions such as asthma, bladder infections, bronchitis, colds, colitis, constipation, Crohn's disease, diarrhea, ear infections, influenza, hemorrhoids, hypertension, irritable bowel syndrome, systemic lupus erythematosis, multiple sclerosis, peptic ulcer, premenstrual syndrome and cramps, pneumonia, prostate enlargement, psoriasis, Raynauds disease, and varicose veins.

Constitutional hydrotherapy consists of a combination of alternating hot and cold treatments to the trunk, front and back of the body. By changing the body temperature using hot and cold towels, you may be able to stimulate the immune system, promote internal healing, detoxify the body and generally improve the circulation.

To perform the treatment:

With Assistance:

1. Place a towel on the floor.
2. Have the person undress from the waist up and lie on the towel, face up.
3. Prepare two moist hot towels (not scalding), wring out and place over chest and abdomen; each towel should be folded in half, resulting in four layered folds.
4. Cover person in blankets to keep warm by retaining heat, (leave in place for five minutes.
5. Apply one thin cold towel on top of hot towels and flip towels; Remove hot towels. Again, cover person with the blanket to keep warm.
6. Leave cold towel on affected area for ten minutes, or until towel becomes warm.
7. Turn person onto their stomach.

8. Repeat the process from step 3, on the back and buttocks.

If there is no one to assist, the single person modification may be performed as follows:

Without Assistance:

1. Prepare a cold towel by soaking in iced water.
2. Take a hot bath or shower for five minutes.
3. Get out and dry off quickly, keeping as warm as possible.
4. Wring out towel which has been soaking in cold or icy water, and wrap it around the trunk of your body.
5. Lie down and cover yourself with a warm blanket.
6. Leave cold towel in place for twenty minutes or until warmed.

Note: It is important never to remove cold towel before it is warmed, or treatment may be ineffective!

Contraindications for use include:
1. Acute bladder infection.
2. Acute asthma.
3. High fever.
4. Pregnancy.

Hot and cold showers
(alternative to hydrotherapy)

Traditionally used for: muscle spasms; encourage blood flow, stimulate immune system, and stimulate nervous system.

Start by taking a hot shower and follow by two minutes of cold shower. Cold water can be worked up to gradually by beginning with cool water and slowly making it colder.

+Understanding homeopathic dosages

Sublingual homeopathic remedies come in a variety of strengths. According to standard homeopathic guidelines, the most dilute is the strongest. The letters X and C indicate the potency. X indicates that the mother tincture has been diluted 1 part in 10. C is diluted 1 part in 100. The number before the X or C indicates how many times the solution was diluted.
Example:
6X = diluted six times to 1 part in 10
12C = diluted twelve times to 1 part in 100
The 12C is more potent

+Product Manufacturers

Supplements:

-Nature's Path, *(vitamins, trace-minerals, ionic silver, herbal skin spray, whole food supplements)* P.O. Box 7862, Venice, FL 34287-7862 (800) 326-5772 www.naturespathinc.com

-Natural Factors *(full line of supplements)* Burnaby, B.C., Canada (800) 322-8704

-Prozyme, *(organic digestive plant enzymes)*, 6444 N. Ridgeway, Lincolnwood, IL 60712 (800) 522-5537

Herbal:

-Natural Labs Corp., *(herbal and flower tinctures)* P.O. Box 5351, Lake Montezuma, AZ 86342 (800) 233-0810 www.alternatehealth.net

-Dr. Christopher's *(herbal products, black ointment, and first aid kits)* 1187, South 1480 West, Orem, UT 84058 (800) 453-1406

-Long Life Catalog, *(Rhododendron caucasicum)* P.O. Box 968 Venice, FL 34275 (888) NATURE-1 email: safes@webtv.net

-Gold Mountain Trading (*velvet antler*), P.O. Box 267, Katikati, Bay of Plenty, New Zealand 64-7-549-3492

-Wakunaga of America (*aged garlic extract*) 23501 Madero, Mission Viejo, CA 91691 (800) 825-7888

Homeopathic:

-Hylands, Inc., Standard Homeopathic Co., *(homeopathic remedies, first aid kits)* P.O. Box 61067, Los Angeles CA 90061 (800) 624-9659 www.hylands.com

-Boiron, *(homeopathic remedies)* 6 Campus Blvd., Newtown Square, PA 19073 (800) BOIRON-1

INDEX

M-N-O-P

R-S-T

V-Z

Valerian, 41, 45, 57, 59
Velvet antler, 17, 19, 77, 79
virus, 18, 28
Vitamin B, 41, 43, 57, 58,
61, 62, 63
Vitamin B$_3$, 57, 58
Vitamin C, 9, 10, 17, 18,
25, 26, 69, 70
Vitamin E, 25, 26

water, 12, 14, 15, 18, 20,
26, 27, 34, 37, 38, 39,
45, 48, 52, 56, 59, 72,
80, 83, 85, 87, 88, 89,
92, 93
water-on-the-knee, 84
White Willow, 41
wounds, 5, 7, 26, 27, 30
Zinc, 17, 19, 25, 26, 61,
63, 69, 71

Bibliography

-Davidson, Alison, Velvet Antler,7/2000, New Century Publishers 2000, Markham, ON

-Dewey, Laurel, The Humorous Herbalist, 1996, Safe Goods, E. Canaan, CT

-Dewey, Laurel, Plant Power, 1999,Safe Goods, E. Canaan, CT

-Page, Linda Rector, Natural Healing, 1996, Healthy Healing Publications, CA

-The complete Book of Vitamin Cures, 1998, Prevention Health Books, Rodale Press, Emmaus, PA

- Ramazanov, Dr. Zakir, Dr. Maria del Mar Bernal Suarez, Effective Natural Stress and Weight Management using Rhodiola rosea and Rhododenron caucasicum, 1999, Safe Goods,
E Canaan, CT

Other Books from
New Century Publishers 2000

Velvet Antler $ 9.95 US
Nature's Superior Tonic $ 14.95 CA

The Fitness for Golfers Handbook $12.95 US
Taking your golf game to the next level. $ 19.95 CA

Self-Care Anywhere $19.95 US
Powerful natural remedies for $ 29.95 CA
common health ailments

Nutritional Leverage for Great Golf $ 9.95 US
How to improve your score on the back nine $ 14.95 CA

To order contact:
(877) 742-7078 toll free
(905) 471-7885

AUTHORS:

Dr. Michael Gazsi, Naturopathic Physician is a graduate of the National College of Naturopathic Medicine in Portland, Oregon. He is medical director of the Center for Integrative Medicine in Ridgefield, Connecticut and is a frequent lecturer on health and nutrition. His articles on alternative medicine have been published in many health magazines, and he is co-author of *Self-Care Anywhere*.

Nina Anderson is an ISSA-certified, Specialist in Performance Nutrition and author of fourteen books on health, aviation safety and sports nutrition. She is a frequent lecturer, radio and television personality and is a contributing editor to several magazines including *Healthy and Natural*, where she writes a monthly column on pet health.